LOW POT.

Diet Cookt

SENIORS

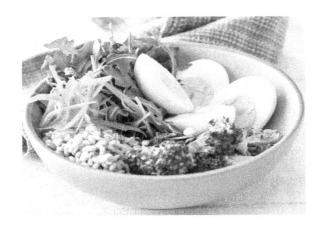

"70 Nutritious Recipes with a Meal Plan to Manage CKD and Hyperkalemia"

Dayna G. Murphy

To Have Access to Other Titles by the Author, Scan me:

Table of Contents

INTRODUCTION

This cookbook was inspired by the amazing experiences of seniors who found vigor and well-being through the transformative power of a low-potassium diet. These resilient individuals began on a journey toward healthy living, embracing flavorful meals tailored to their personal nutritional requirements. This cookbook was inspired by their increased energy, enhanced kidney function, and overall health. Despite dietary constraints, their commitment to enjoy life to the fullest emphasized the value of culinary innovation and conscious nutrition. Each recipe in these pages is a tribute to the seniors who welcomed change and discovered joy in the kitchen. Their experiences highlight the possibility of delicious, low-potassium options that not only maintain health but also celebrate the joys of sharing healthful meals with loved ones. May their experiences inspire others to pursue their own paths to fitness, resilience, and the joy of delicious eating.

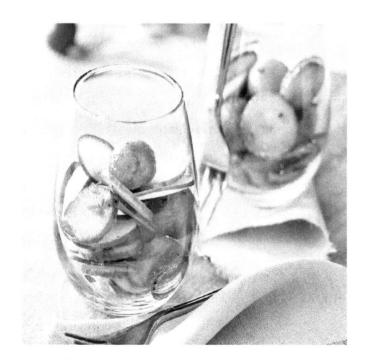

CHAPTER 1

Understanding Potassium

Potassium's Dietary Importance

Potassium is an essential mineral that is required for the normal functioning of many body systems. Seniors, like people of all ages, require an appropriate potassium consumption for good health. Potassium has several important roles, including:

1. **Electrolyte Balance:** Potassium is an electrolyte that, along with sodium, regulates the fluid balance in and out of cells. This is essential for appropriate hydration and supporting cellular functioning.

2. **Heart Health:** Potassium is believed to aid in the regulation of cardiac rhythm and contribute to overall cardiovascular health. Adequate potassium intake may help lower

blood pressure, reduce the risk of strokes, and support the effective functioning of the heart muscle.

3. Muscle Contractions: Potassium is required for muscular contraction, especially smooth muscle contraction in the digestive system. It aids in the prevention of muscle cramps and the maintenance of muscular strength.

4. Nervous System Function: Potassium is involved in the transmission of nerve impulses in the nervous system. A healthy potassium level promotes normal nerve cell communication, which improves cognitive function and overall neurological health.

Potassium Intake Risks for Seniors

While potassium is essential for health, high quantities, particularly in the elderly, can be dangerous. Seniors may be more prone to kidney function decrease, and reduced kidney function can have an impact on the body's capacity to manage potassium. High potassium intake is connected with the following risks:

- **Renal Dysfunction:** Seniors with impaired renal function may have difficulty excreting excess potassium. High potassium levels can cause hyperkalemia, a kidney-related illness that can cause lethargy, irregular heartbeats, and other serious issues.

- **Cardiac Complications:** Excess potassium can disturb the heart's natural rhythm, causing palpitations, arrhythmias, or even cardiac collapse. Seniors, especially those with pre-existing heart issues, must exercise caution when it comes to potassium balance.

Advantages of a Low Potassium Diet

Adopting a low potassium diet can provide various benefits for seniors who are struggling with kidney function or other health issues:

Kidney Health: A low potassium diet helps control potassium levels, minimizing the burden on kidneys that are already damaged. This can help to decrease the progression of renal disease and improve symptoms.

- **Heart Health:** Seniors with cardiovascular difficulties may benefit from a low potassium diet since it promotes overall heart health by supporting a steady heart rhythm and lowering the risk of excessive blood pressure.

- **Symptom Management:** People who have symptoms connected to excessive potassium levels, such as muscle weakness, fatigue, or irregular heartbeats, may benefit from a low potassium diet that is properly monitored.

CHAPTER 2

Basics of a Low Potassium Diet

Identifying Potassium-Rich Foods

Identification of high-potassium foods is critical for seniors on a low-potassium diet. While potassium is an essential nutrient, people with certain health concerns, such as kidney disease, may need to watch their potassium consumption more strictly. Here's a list of high-potassium foods from each food group:

Fruits:

Certain fruits are high in potassium, and elders should limit their intake. Fruits that are high in potassium include:

- **Bananas:** A popular fruit known for its potassium content, bananas should be consumed in moderation.

- **Oranges and orange juice:** Citrus fruits are high in vitamin C, but they are also high in potassium. Berries, for example, have a lower potassium concentration than other fruits.
- **Cantaloupe:** This sweet melon is delightful, but it is high in potassium.
- **Kiwi:** Although a nutritious fruit, kiwi is high in potassium and should be consumed in moderation.

Vegetables:

Vegetables are important components of a healthy diet, although certain varieties are higher in potassium than others. Seniors should exercise caution when dealing with the following:

- **Potatoes:** Potatoes are high in potassium whether baked, mashed, or fried. Consider sweet potatoes as a lower-potassium alternative.
- **Tomatoes and Tomato goods:** Potassium is found in tomatoes, tomato

sauce, and tomato-based goods. Choose low-potassium vegetables for sauces and salads.

- **Spinach:** Spinach, a nutrient-dense leafy green, is high in potassium. Other greens to try include kale and lettuce.

Dairy:

Dairy products are high in calcium, but they also contain potassium. Seniors should limit their consumption of high-potassium dairy products such as:

- **Milk:** Cow's milk is high in calcium but low in potassium. Consider alternatives with reduced potassium levels, such as almond or rice milk.
- **Yogurt:** Some yogurts, particularly Greek yogurt, contain a lot of potassium. Choose yogurt with a reduced potassium concentration.
- **Cheese:** Certain cheeses, such as Swiss and cheddar, contain significant

amounts of potassium. Choose cheeses with reduced potassium levels.

Proteins:

Protein-rich diets, particularly animal proteins, can help you get enough potassium. Seniors should be careful of the potassium content of the foods listed below:

- **Fish:** Potassium is abundant in certain species of fish, such as salmon and tuna. Look into low-potassium fish like tilapia or cod.

- **Chicken:** Despite being a lean protein, chicken includes potassium. Portion amounts should be adjusted, and alternate protein sources should be considered.

- **Red meats:** Beef, pork, and lamb are high in both protein and potassium. Moderation and lean cuts are essential.

Cereals:

Grains can also increase potassium levels, and seniors should be aware of the following potassium-rich foods:

- **Whole Grains:** Whole wheat, brown rice, and quinoa are all high in potassium. Consider adopting smaller servings or experimenting with low-potassium cereals such as white rice.

Beverages:

While hydrated, certain beverages might contribute to potassium consumption. Seniors should be aware of the following:

- **Sports Drinks:** Sports drinks may contain potassium supplements. Choose water or drinks designed expressly for people on a low-potassium diet.
- **Fruit liquids:** Even 100% fruit juices might contain a lot of potassium. Choose potassium-free alternatives such as apple or cranberry juice.

Seniors can make smart dietary decisions to regulate their potassium intake by being aware of high-potassium items within each category. Working with a healthcare expert or a certified dietitian to develop a specific low potassium diet plan based on individual health needs is recommended.

Understanding Food Labels

For seniors on a low potassium diet, knowing how to read food labels is critical. Food labels provide important information regarding the nutrient content of packaged goods, allowing consumers to make more educated decisions. Here is a breakdown of major factors to consider while reading food labels:

1. Potassium and Sodium Content

Seniors should pay close attention to the salt and potassium content on food labels. While potassium is the primary focus for those on a low potassium diet, salt intake is also crucial, especially for people who are trying to lose weight. Consider the following suggestions:

- **Examine the Serving Size:** Keep in mind the serving size specified on the label. The nutritional amount is frequently stated per serving, therefore eating numerous portions can dramatically increase potassium intake.

- **Look for Potassium Content:** Determine the amount of potassium in each serving. Foods labeled "low potassium" often contain 150 mg of potassium or less per serving.

- **Assess Sodium Levels:** In addition to potassium, consider sodium content. High salt intake can contribute to fluid retention and have a bad impact on cardiovascular health.

- **Compare Nutrient Content of Similar Products:** When deciding between similar products, compare their nutrient content. Choose goods with lower levels of potassium and sodium.

2. Potassium Sources Unknown

Certain foods may contain potassium sources that are not immediately evident. Seniors should be on the lookout for and manage these hidden potassium sources:

- **Preservatives and additives:** Potassium is found in some food additives such as potassium chloride, potassium citrate, and monopotassium phosphate. These compounds are frequently used to enhance flavor or as preservatives.

- **Processed Foods:** Potassium is hidden in many processed and convenience foods. Check the labels of canned soups, pre-packaged meals, and frozen entrees for additional potassium.

- **Baked Foods:** Bread, cakes, and pastries may include potassium-based additions. Consider making your own or purchasing specially prepared low-potassium alternatives.

- **Condiments and sauces:** Certain condiments and sauces, such as soy sauce, barbecue sauce, and ketchup, can be high in potassium. Look for alternatives that are low in salt and potassium, or use them sparingly.

- **Snack Foods:** Preservatives in potato chips, pretzels, and other snacks may include potassium. Consider low-potassium snacks such as air-popped popcorn or rice cakes.

- **Dietary Supplements:** Potassium may be included in some dietary supplements. Before taking any supplements, seniors with certain dietary limitations should contact with a healthcare provider.

CHAPTER 3

Planning Low Potassium Meals

Meal Planning Techniques

A good low-potassium diet for seniors begins with effective meal planning. Individuals can enjoy a range of delicious and nutritious meals while controlling their potassium intake by applying smart measures. Here are some important meal planning strategies:

1. Portion Management

Controlling potassium intake begins with portion control. Seniors can have a healthy diet without exceeding their dietary limitations by being cautious of serving sizes. Consider the following suggestions:

- **Use Measuring Tools:** To correctly portion out ingredients, use measuring cups and scales. This is especially crucial for potassium-rich foods such as fruits, vegetables, and cereals.

- **Balance Nutrients:** Make sure each meal contains a good mix of macronutrients (carbohydrates, proteins, and fats). This helps to maintain total nutrition while providing a sense of fulfillment.

- **Divide Meals into Smaller Portions:** Instead of eating huge meals throughout the day, consider eating smaller, more frequent meals throughout the day. This can help to more equally divide potassium intake.

- **Choose Low-Potassium Substitutes:** Choose low-potassium substitutes or lesser quantities of high-potassium foods. Replace a typical banana, for example, with a smaller, less ripe banana.

2. Cooking Techniques

The manner food is prepared can have a big impact on its potassium concentration. To control potassium levels in their meals, seniors can use the following cooking methods:

- **Soaking and boiling:** Soaking and boiling vegetables and legumes can reduce their potassium levels. Consider utilizing a double-cooking method, in which vegetables are first cooked and then the water is discarded before further cooking.

- **Steaming:** Steaming is a mild cooking method that helps nutrients retain while avoiding potassium loss. It is especially beneficial on veggies.

- **Grilling and Roasting:** Grilling and roasting provide flavor without the use of high-potassium foods. Instead of high-potassium sauces, season with herbs and spices.

- **Sauteing with Olive Oil:** Sauteing with olive oil enhances taste without drastically boosting potassium levels.
- **Avoid Using High-Potassium Cooking Ingredients:** Avoid using high-potassium cooking ingredients, such as tomato-based sauces. Instead, try out low-potassium alternatives or various flavor characteristics.

3. Frequency of Meals

Meal frequency contributes to potassium intake management and overall well-being. Seniors can maximize their meal frequency by taking the following factors into account:

- **Meals:** Aim for three well-balanced meals every day to give a consistent source of nutrients. Each meal should include a range of low-potassium foods.
- **nutritious Snacking:** Include nutritious snacks between meals to minimize

feeling hungry and overeating during big meals. Choose snacks that adhere to low-potassium requirements.

- **Hydration:** Drink plenty of water throughout the day to stay hydrated. Adequate hydration is vital for kidney function and can help regulate potassium levels.

- **Consult a Dietitian:** Work with a qualified dietitian to develop a meal plan that meets your specific nutritional needs and interests. A tailored strategy ensures that dietary needs are satisfied while potassium intake is managed.

Sample Meal Plans

Creating well-balanced and appealing meal plans is crucial for seniors following a low-potassium diet. Here are sample meal plans for breakfast, lunch, dinner, and snacks:

Breakfast

Option 1:

- Scrambled Eggs with Fresh Herbs (parsley, chives)
- Whole Grain Toast (white bread or low-potassium alternative)
- Sliced Melon (cantaloupe or honeydew)

Option 2:

- Greek Yogurt Parfait with Low-Potassium Fruits (berries, apple)
- Granola (low-potassium option)
- Sprinkle of Chopped Nuts (in moderation)

Option 3:

- Oatmeal (made with water or low-potassium milk substitute)
- Sliced Banana (in moderation)
- Almond Butter (small portion)

Lunch

Option 1:

- Grilled Chicken Salad with Mixed Greens (lettuce, arugula)
- Cherry Tomatoes and Cucumbers
- Quinoa (cooked and cooled)
- Olive Oil and Balsamic Vinegar Dressing

Option 2:

- Turkey and Avocado Wrap (using a low-potassium tortilla)
- Carrot Sticks
- Fresh Berries (strawberries, blueberries)

Option 3:

- Lentil Soup (homemade with low-potassium vegetables)
- Whole Grain Crackers (low-potassium option)
- Sliced Pear (in moderation)

Dinner

Option 1:

- Baked Salmon with Lemon and Dill
- Mashed Cauliflower (instead of potatoes)
- Steamed Green Beans
- Quinoa Pilaf

Option 2:

- Stir-Fried Tofu with Broccoli and Bell Peppers
- Brown Rice (portion-controlled)
- Sliced Mango (in moderation)

Option 3:

- Grilled Shrimp Skewers
- Zucchini Noodles (zoodles)
- Roasted Asparagus
- Wild Rice (portion-controlled)

Snacks

Option 1:

- Air-Popped Popcorn (sprinkled with herbs, not salt)
- Fresh Fruit Salad (low-potassium fruits)

Option 2:

- Greek Yogurt (low-potassium)
- Handful of Almonds (portion-controlled)
- Sliced Peach (in moderation)

Option 3:

- Rice Cakes with Hummus
- Celery Sticks
- Diced Pineapple (in moderation)

CHAPTER 4

Delicious and Nutritious Recipes and How to Prepare Them

10 Breakfast Recipes

1. Spinach and Feta Scrambled Eggs

Ingredients:

- 2 eggs
- 1/4 cup chopped fresh spinach
- 1 tablespoon crumbled feta cheese
- Season with salt and pepper to taste

Instructions:

1. In a mixing basin, whisk the eggs until completely combined.

2. Melt butter in a nonstick skillet over medium heat.

3. Cook the chopped spinach in the skillet until wilted.

4. Gently pour the beaten eggs into the skillet.

5. Cook the eggs until they are scrambled and cooked to your satisfaction.

6. Top with feta cheese and season with salt and pepper.

Preparation Time: 10 minutes

2. Chia Seed Pudding Overnight

Ingredients:

- 2 teaspoons chia seeds
- 1/2 cup almond milk (or other low-potassium milk alternative)
- 1 teaspoon honey
- 1/4 teaspoon vanilla extract
- Fresh berries for garnish

Instructions:

1. Combine chia seeds, almond milk, vanilla essence, and honey in a mixing dish.

2. Stir well and place in the refrigerator overnight.

3. Before serving, top with fresh berries in the morning.

Preparation Time: 5 minutes (including overnight chilling)

3. Smoothie with bananas and almond butter

Ingredients:

- 1 banana, ripe
- 1 tbsp. almond butter
- 1/2 cup low-potassium milk substitute (rice milk, for example)
- Optional (ice cubes)

Instructions:

1. Combine the banana, almond butter, and milk substitute in a blender.

2. Puree until smooth.

3. If desired, add ice cubes and mix again.

4. Strain into a glass and serve.

Preparation Time: 5 minutes

4. Pineapple Cottage Cheese

Ingredients:

- 1/2 cup cottage cheese (low-fat)
- 1/2 cup chopped fresh pineapple

Instructions:

1. Place the cottage cheese in a mixing basin.

2. Garnish with diced pineapple.

3. Gently combine and serve.

Preparation Time: 5 minutes

5. Breakfast Wrap with Avocado and Tomato

Ingredients:

- 1 whole-grain (low-potassium) tortilla
- half an avocado, sliced
- 1 tiny sliced tomato
- Chopped fresh cilantro

Instructions:

1. Spread the tortilla out flat.

2. In the center, arrange avocado slices and sliced tomatoes.

3. Garnish with cilantro, if desired.

4. Fold the tortilla in half and make it into a wrap.

Preparation Time: 8 minutes

6. Pancakes with Blueberries and Oats

Ingredients:

- 1/2 cup coarsely ground oats
- 1/2 mashed banana
- 1/4 cup fresh blueberries
- 1/4 cup low-potassium milk alternative
- 1 tablespoon baking powder

Instructions:

1. Combine oat flour, mashed banana, blueberries, milk substitute, and baking powder in a mixing dish.

2. Combine until thoroughly blended.

3. Heat a nonstick frying pan and pour batter into it to make little pancakes.

4. Cook until surface bubbles appear, then flip and cook the other side.

Preparation Time: 15 Minutes

7. Apple Cinnamon Quinoa Bowl

Ingredients:

- 1/2 cup cooked quinoa
- 1 tiny chopped apple
- 1/4 tsp cinnamon

- 1 tablespoon walnuts, chopped

Instructions:

1. Combine cooked quinoa, diced apple, and cinnamon in a mixing bowl.

2. Garnish with chopped walnuts.

3. Combine all of the ingredients and serve.

Preparation Time: 10 minutes (if quinoa is already cooked)

8. Greek Yogurt and Berries Parfait

Ingredients:

- 1/2 cup Greek yogurt (low in potassium)
- 1/4 cup low-potassium granola
- Berries (strawberries and blueberries)

Instructions:

1. Layer Greek yogurt, granola, and fresh berries in a glass.

2. Continue layering.

3. Garnish with additional berries.

Preparation Time: 5 minutes

9. Spinach and Tomato Omelette

Ingredients:

- 2 eggs
- A handful of chopped fresh spinach
- 1 small sliced tomato
- Salt and pepper to taste

Instructions:

1. In a mixing basin, whisk the eggs.

2. Melt butter in a nonstick skillet over medium heat.

3. Cook until the spinach and tomatoes are wilted in the skillet.

4. Scatter the vegetables with the beaten eggs.

5. Cook until the eggs are set, folding the omelette in half halfway through.

Preparation Time: 10 minutes

10. Rice Cake with Almond Butter and Strawberries

Ingredients:

- 1 low-potassium rice cake
- 1 tbsp. almond butter
- Sliced fresh strawberries

Instructions:

1. Spread the almond butter on top of the rice cake.

2. Garnish with strawberries, if desired.

3. Enjoy this quick and easy snack.

Preparation Time: 5 minutes

10 Lunch Recipes

1. Salad with grilled chicken and quinoa

Ingredients:

- 1 cup quinoa, cooked
- sliced grilled chicken breast
- Salad greens (lettuce and arugula)
- Dressing: cherry tomatoes, half olive oil, and balsamic vinegar

Instructions:

1. Combine the quinoa, grilled chicken, salad greens, and cherry tomatoes in a mixing bowl.

2. Dressing: drizzle with olive oil and balsamic vinegar.

3. Gently toss and serve.

Prep Time: 20 minutes (if quinoa and chicken are cooked ahead of time)

2. Wrap with Turkey and Avocado

Ingredients:

- turkey breast, sliced
- Whole-grain (low-potassium) tortilla
- sliced ripe avocado
- Lettuce leaves, fresh

Instructions:

1. Arrange turkey pieces, avocado, and lettuce on a flat tortilla.
2. Make a wrap with the tortilla.
3. Serve cut in half.

Preparation Time: 10 minutes

3. Soup with lentils and vegetables

Ingredients:

- 1 cooked cup lentils
- Vegetables (carrots, celery, and zucchini)
- Broth de légumes à faible teneur en sodium

- Spices and herbs (thyme, oregano)
- Cooking with olive oil

Instructions:

1. Cook until the vegetables are softened in olive oil.

2. Pour in the cooked lentils and vegetable broth.

3. Season with herbs and spices to taste.

4. Simmer until the flavors combine and the vegetables are soft.

Time to prepare: 30 minutes (if lentils are pre-cooked)

4. Bowl of Quinoa with Roasted Vegetables

Ingredients:

- 1 cup quinoa, cooked
- Roasted vegetables (bell peppers, eggplant, and zucchini)
- Dressing of olive oil and lemon
- chopped fresh parsley

Instructions:

1. Toss cooked quinoa with roasted veggies.

2. Dress with olive oil and lemon juice.

3. Garnish with fresh parsley, if desired.

Time to prepare: 25 minutes (if quinoa is pre-cooked)

5. Lettuce Wraps with Tuna Salad

Ingredients:

- Tuna with water, drained Greek yogurt (low in potassium)
- Celery and red onion, diced
- Wrapping lettuce leaves

Instructions:

1. Combine tuna, Greek yogurt, celery, and red onion in a mixing bowl.

2. Fill lettuce leaves with tuna salad.

3. Wrap the leaves with lettuce leaves and serve.

Preparation Time: 15 minutes

6. Salad with Chickpeas and Cucumbers

Ingredients:

- Chickpeas, cucumber, chopped cherry tomatoes, half olive oil, and lemon dressing
- Mint, fresh, chopped

Instructions:

1. In a mixing dish, combine chickpeas, cucumber, and cherry tomatoes.

2. Dress with olive oil and lemon juice.

3. Garnish with fresh mint, if desired.

Preparation Time: 15 minutes

7. Lemon and Dill Baked Salmon

Ingredients:

- Fillet of salmon
- Lemon wedges
- Olive oil, chopped fresh dill
- Season with salt and pepper to taste.

Instructions:

1. Arrange the fish on a baking sheet.

2. Season with salt, pepper, and chopped dill and drizzle with olive oil.

3. Serve with lemon slices on top.

4. Bake until the salmon is done.

Preparation Time: 20 minutes

8 Stuffed Bell Peppers with Spinach and Feta

Ingredients:

- halved bell peppers with seeds removed
- Feta cheese, chopped spinach, crumbled
- Optional quinoa
- Spices and herbs (oregano, garlic powder)

Instructions:

1. Preheat the oven to 350°F and roast the bell peppers until soft.

2. Combine chopped spinach, feta cheese, and cooked quinoa (if using) in a mixing bowl.

3. Fill the bell peppers halfway with the spinach-feta mixture.

4. Bake until the filling is well cooked.

Preparation Time: 30 minutes (if quinoa is already cooked)

9. Stir-Fry with Chicken and Vegetables

Ingredients:

- thinly sliced chicken breast
- Vegetable stir-fry (broccoli, bell peppers, snap peas)
- Soy sauce with low sodium
- Sesame seed oil
- Brown rice (restricted portion)

Instructions:

1. Cook chicken slices in sesame oil until done.

2. Continue to stir-fry the mixed vegetables.

3. Add the low-sodium soy sauce.

4. Over portion-controlled brown rice, serve.

Preparation Time: 20 minutes

10. Lettuce Wraps with Egg Salad

Ingredients:

- Hard-boiled eggs, low-potassium Greek yogurt
- Celery and green onion, diced
- Wrapping lettuce leaves

Instructions:

1. Combine hard-boiled eggs, Greek yogurt, celery, and green onion in a mixing bowl.

2. Fill lettuce leaves with the egg salad.

3. Wrap the leaves with lettuce leaves and serve.

Preparation Time: 15 minutes

10 Dinner Recipes

1. Lemon Herb Baked Chicken

Ingredients:

- Chicken thighs or breasts
- Lemon juice, freshly squeezed
- Minced garlic
- Olive oil - Fresh herbs (thyme, rosemary)
- Season with salt and pepper to taste

Instructions:

1. Preheat the oven to 350°F and place the chicken in a baking dish.

2. To make a marinade, combine lemon juice, minced garlic, fresh herbs, and olive oil.

3. Drizzle the marinade over the chicken and season with salt & pepper to taste.

4. Bake until the chicken is thoroughly done.

Preparation Time: 25 minutes

2. Stuffed Peppers with Quinoa and Vegetables

Ingredients:

- Halved bell peppers with seeds removed - Cooked quinoa
- Vegetable mixture (zucchini, tomatoes, corn)
- Extra virgin olive oil
- Spices and herbs (cumin, paprika)

Instructions:

1. Preheat the oven to 350°F and roast the bell peppers until soft.

2. Combine cooked quinoa, mixed vegetables, olive oil, and herbs in a mixing bowl.

3. Stuff the quinoa and veggie mixture into the bell peppers.

4. Bake until the filling is thoroughly cooked.

Preparation Time: 30 minutes (if quinoa is already cooked)

3. Grilled Salmon with Dill Sauce

Ingredients:

- Salmon fillet
- Fresh dill, diced
- Low-potassium Greek yogurt
- Fresh lemon juice
- Extra virgin olive oil
- Season with salt and pepper to taste

Instructions:

1. Preheat the grill to high heat and spray the salmon with olive oil.

2. Grill the salmon until it is cooked through.

3. To make the sauce, combine chopped dill, Greek yogurt, and lemon juice in a mixing dish.

4. Drizzle the dill sauce over the grilled fish.

Preparation Time: 20 minutes

4. Stir-Fry of Lentils and Vegetables

Ingredients:

- Cooked lentils
- Vegetable stir-fry mix (broccoli, bell peppers, snap peas)
- Soy sauce with low sodium
- Sesame seed oil
- Portion-controlled brown rice

Instructions:

1. Heat sesame oil in a skillet and stir-fry cooked lentils and mixed vegetables.

2. Stir in the low-sodium soy sauce.

3. Arrange on a bed of portion-controlled brown rice.

Preparation Time: 20 minutes (if lentils are already cooked)

5. Pesto Zucchini Noodles

Ingredients:

- Spiralized zucchini
- Homemade or store-bought pesto (low potassium)
- Halved cherry tomatoes

- Pine nuts for garnish

Instructions:

1. Spiralize the zucchini to make noodles.

2. Cook zucchini noodles in a pan until just soft.

3. Combine pesto and cherry tomatoes in a mixing bowl.

4. Garnish with pine nuts before serving.

Preparation Time: 15 Minutes

6. Skewers of chicken and vegetables

Ingredients:

- Cubed chicken breast
- Peppers, onions, and cherry tomatoes
- A marinade of olive oil and lemon juice
- Spices and herbs (rosemary, thyme)
- Quinoa (in moderation)

Instructions:

1. Skewer the chicken and vegetables.

2. For the marinade, combine olive oil, lemon juice, herbs, and spices.

3. Grill the skewers until the chicken is thoroughly cooked.

4. Top with portion-controlled quinoa.

Preparation Time: 30 minutes (if quinoa is already cooked)

7. Risotto with Spinach and Mushrooms

Ingredients:

- Arborio rice
- Chopped fresh spinach
- Sliced mushrooms
- Vegetable broth with low sodium
- Parmesan cheese (optional)
- Olive oil

Instructions:

1. Sauté mushrooms in olive oil in a pan.

2. Stir in the Arborio rice until it is lightly browned.

3. Stir in the vegetable broth gradually until the rice is tender.

4. Fold in the spinach and, if preferred, the Parmesan cheese.

Preparation Time: 40 minutes

8. Stir-Fried Shrimp with Asparagus

Ingredients:

- Peeled and deveined shrimp
- Trimmed fresh asparagus
- Low-sodium soy sauce
- Minced garlic
- Sesame seed oil
- Portion-controlled brown rice

Instructions:

1. Cook the shrimp and asparagus in sesame oil until they are done.

2. Stir in the minced garlic and low-sodium soy sauce.

3. Arrange on a bed of portion-controlled brown rice.

Preparation Time: 25 minutes (if rice is already cooked)

9. Baked Eggplant with Tomato

Ingredients:

- Sliced eggplant
- Sliced fresh tomatoes
- Extra virgin olive oil
- Herbs and spices (oregano, basil)
- Optional mozzarella cheese

Instructions:

1. Preheat the oven to 350°F and line a baking dish with eggplant and tomato slices.

2. Drizzle with olive oil and top with fresh herbs.

3. If desired, top with mozzarella cheese.

4. Bake the vegetables until they are soft.

Preparation Time: 30 minutes

10. Turkey and Sweet Potato Hash

Ingredients:

- Ground turkey
- Diced sweet potatoes
- Diced onion
- Minced garlic
- Spices and herbs (paprika, thyme)
- Olive oil

Instructions:

1. Brown ground turkey in olive oil in a skillet.

2. Stir in the cubed sweet potatoes, onion, and garlic.

3. Add herbs and spices to taste.

4. Continue to cook until the sweet potatoes are soft.

Preparation Time: 30 minutes

10 Appetizers and Snacks

1. Platter of Hummus and Veggies

Ingredients:

- Hummus with low potassium
- Carrot sticks
- Cucumber slices
- Bell pepper strips

Instructions:

1. Arrange on a tray carrot sticks, cucumber slices, and bell pepper strips.

2. Serve with low-potassium hummus on the side for dipping.

Preparation Time: 10 minutes

2. Jicama Chips Guacamole

Ingredients:

- One ripe avocado
- Diced tomato
- Finely sliced red onion
- Lime juice
- Jicama cut into chips

Instructions:

1. Mash the avocado and combine it with the diced tomato, red onion, and lime juice.

2. Thinly slice the jicama.

3. Toss guacamole with jicama chips and serve.

Preparation Time: 15 Minutes

3. Greek Yogurt and Berry Parfait

Ingredients:

- Greek yogurt with low potassium
- Strawberries and blueberries mixed

- Low-potassium granola

Instructions:

1. Layer Greek yogurt, mixed berries, and granola in a glass.

2. Continue with the layers.

3. Garnish with additional berries.

Preparation Time: 5 minutes

4. Almond Butter Rice Cake with Banana Slices

Ingredients:

- Low-potassium rice cake
- Almond milk
- Sliced banana

Instructions:

1. Spread the almond butter on top of the rice cake.

2. Garnish with banana slices.

3. Enjoy this quick and easy snack.

Preparation Time: 5 minutes

5. Caprese Skewers

Ingredients:

- Balsamic glaze
- Cherry tomatoes
- Fresh mozzarella balls
- Basil leaves

Instructions:

1. Skewer cherry tomatoes, mozzarella balls, and basil leaves.

2. Before serving, drizzle with balsamic glaze.

Preparation Time: 10 minutes

6. Chickpeas Roasted

Ingredients:

- Drained and washed canned chickpeas
- Olive oil
- Spices and herbs (cumin, paprika)
- Salt

Instructions:

1. Heat the oven to 350°F and toss the chickpeas with the olive oil, herbs, and spices.

2. Arrange the chickpeas on a baking sheet.

3. Roast until crisp, shaking the pan every now and again.

Time to Prepare: 30 minutes (including roasting time)

7. Cups of Cottage Cheese and Pineapple

Ingredients:
- Cottage cheese (low-fat)
- Diced fresh pineapple

Instructions:

1. Divide the cottage cheese into small cups.

2. Sprinkle with chopped fresh pineapple.

3. Serve cold.

Preparation Time: 5 minutes

8. Almond Butter-Sliced Apple

Ingredients:
- Sliced apple
- Almond butter

Instructions:

1. Spread almond butter on slices of apple.

2. Place on a dish and serve.

Preparation Time: 5 minutes

9. Tomato and Avocado Salsa

Ingredients:

- Diced ripe avocado
- Diced tomato
- Diced red onion
- Diced cilantro
- Lime juice

Instructions:

1. Combine chopped avocado, tomato, red onion, cilantro, and lime juice in a mixing dish.

2. Serve with tortilla chips that are low in potassium.

Preparation Time: 10 minutes

10. Smoked Salmon Cucumber Roll-Ups

Ingredients:

- Low-fat cream cheese
- English cucumber, thinly sliced lengthwise
- Salmon smoked

- Dill, fresh

Instructions:

1. On cucumber slices, spread a thin layer of cream cheese.

2. Garnish with smoked salmon and dill.

3. Roll up and use toothpicks to secure.

Preparation Time: 15 Minutes

10 Soups and Salads

1. Soup with Chicken and Vegetables

Ingredients:

- Low-sodium chicken broth
- Shredded cooked chicken breast
- Diced carrots
- Chopped celery
- Sliced zucchini
- chopped fresh parsley
- salt and pepper to taste

Instructions:

1. Bring chicken broth to a simmer in a pot.

2. Stir in the shredded chicken, carrots, celery, and zucchini slices.

3. Cook until the vegetables are soft.

4. Season with salt and pepper to taste, then top with fresh parsley.

Preparation Time: 30 minutes (if chicken is already cooked)

2. Salad with Spinach and Strawberries

Ingredients:

- Fresh spinach leaves
- Sliced strawberries
- Crumbled goat cheese
- Low-potassium balsamic vinaigrette

Instructions:

1. Combine fresh spinach, sliced strawberries, and crumbled goat cheese in a mixing basin.

2. Toss gently with low-potassium balsamic vinaigrette.

Preparation Time 10 minutes

3. Soup with Tomatoes and Basil

Ingredients:

- Low-sodium tomato soup
- Diced fresh tomatoes
- Diced fresh basil
- Olive oil

Instructions:

1. In a pot, heat low-sodium tomato soup.

2. Stir in the diced fresh tomatoes and basil.

3. Cook until the tomatoes are soft.

4. Before serving, drizzle with olive oil.

Preparation Time: 15 Minutes

4. Greek Salad with Grilled Chicken

Ingredients:

- Chopped Romaine lettuce
- Sliced grilled chicken breast
- Diced cucumber
- Halved cherry tomatoes
- Pitted Kalamata olives
- Crumbled Feta cheese
- Greek dressing (low potassium)

Instructions:

1. Toss together lettuce, grilled chicken, cucumber, cherry tomatoes, olives, and feta cheese in a large mixing dish.

2. Toss gently with low-potassium Greek dressing.

Preparation Time: 20 minutes (if chicken is already cooked)

5. Butternut Squash Soup

Ingredients:

- Peeled and diced butternut squash
- Chopped onion
- Vegetable broth (low sodium)
- Ground nutmeg
- Extra virgin olive oil

Instructions:

1. Saute chopped onions in olive oil in a saucepan till transparent.

2. Stir in the butternut squash dices and vegetable broth.

3. Cook until the squash is soft.

4. Blend until smooth, then season with nutmeg powder.

Preparation Time: 30 minutes

6. Salad with Tuna and White Beans

Ingredients:

- Drained canned tuna in water
- rinsed and drained white beans
- finely chopped red onion
- halved cherry tomatoes
- chopped fresh parsley
- olive oil and lemon dressing (low potassium)

Instructions:

1. Combine tuna, white beans, red onion, cherry tomatoes, and parsley in a mixing bowl.
2. Drizzle with lemon dressing and low-potassium olive oil.

Preparation Time: 15 Minutes

7. Soup with Cauliflower and Leek

Ingredients:

- Chopped cauliflower
- Sliced leeks
- Low-sodium vegetable broth
- Minced garlic
- Thyme, fresh
- Extra virgin olive oil

Instructions:

1. In olive oil, sauté sliced leeks and minced garlic until mellow.

2. Stir in the cauliflower and fresh thyme.

3. Add the low-sodium vegetable broth and cook until the cauliflower is soft.

4. Puree until smooth.

Preparation Time: 25 minutes

8. Salad with Shrimp and Avocado

Ingredients:

- Cooked and peeled shrimp
- Diced avocado
- Mixed greens (arugula, spinach)
- Halved cherry tomatoes
- Cilantro, diced

- Lime vinaigrette (low potassium)

Instructions:

1. Combine cooked shrimp, diced avocado, mixed greens, cherry tomatoes, and cilantro in a mixing dish.

2. Drizzle with lime vinaigrette with low potassium.

Preparation Time: 15 Minutes

9.Potato Leek Soup

Ingredients:

- Peeled and chopped potatoes
- Sliced leeks
- Low-sodium chicken or veggie broth
- Fresh or dried thyme
- Olive oil

Instructions:

1. In a skillet, sauté sliced leeks in olive oil until softened.

2. Combine diced potatoes, thyme, and low-sodium broth in a mixing bowl.

3. Cook until the potatoes are soft.

4. Puree until smooth.

Preparation Time: 30 minutes

10. Salad with Cucumber and Dill

Ingredients:

- Thinly sliced cucumbers
- Low-fat Greek yogurt
- Fresh dill, diced
- Thinly sliced red onion
- Salt and pepper to taste

Instructions:

1. Combine thinly sliced cucumbers, low-fat Greek yogurt, chopped dill, and thinly sliced red onion in a mixing dish.

2. Season with salt and pepper to taste.

Preparation Time: 10 minutes

10 Desserts

1. Apples Baked with Cinnamon and Walnuts

Ingredients:

- Cored and halved apples

- Ground cinnamon
- Chopped walnuts
- Optional: honey

Instructions:

1. Preheat the oven to 350°F and arrange the cored and halved apples in a baking dish.

2. Garnish with ground cinnamon and walnuts.

3. If desired, drizzle with honey.

4. Bake until the apples are soft.

Preparation Time: 20 minutes

2. Banana Ice Cream

Ingredients:

- Sliced and frozen ripe bananas
- Vanilla extract (optional)
- Toppings with low potassium (such as chopped nuts or berries)

Instructions:

1. Puree frozen banana slices till smooth.

2. If desired, add vanilla extract.

3. Spoon into dishes and garnish with low-potassium alternatives.

Preparation Time: 10 minutes

3. Whipped Cream Berry Parfait

Ingredients:

- Strawberries and blueberries mixed
- Whipped cream with a low potassium content
- Optional crushed low-potassium cookies

Instructions:

1. Layer mixed berries and low-potassium whipped cream in a glass.

2. Continue layering.

3. If desired, top with crushed low-potassium cookies.

Preparation Time: 10 minutes

4. Peach Sorbet

Ingredients:

- Peaches, frozen
- Lemon juice
- Optional: honey

Instructions:

1. In a blender, combine frozen peaches and lemon juice until smooth.

2. If preferred, add honey for sweetness.

3. Freeze until hard, or serve right now.

Preparation Time: 15 Minute

5. Cinnamon Rice Pudding

Ingredients:

- Cooked white rice
- Milk substitute with low potassium (e.g., rice milk)
- Cinnamon powder
- Optional sugar

Instructions:

1. Combine cooked rice, low-potassium milk substitute, and ground cinnamon in a saucepan.

2. Cook until creamy over low heat.

3. If desired, add sugar.

4. Allow to cool before serving.

Preparation Time: 25 minutes (if rice is already cooked)

6. Salad with Watermelon and Mint

Ingredients:

- Cubed watermelon
- Chopped fresh mint
- Lime juice

Instructions:

1. Combine cubed watermelon and chopped fresh mint in a mixing basin.

2. Garnish with lime juice.

3. Gently toss and chill before serving.

Preparation Time: 10 minutes

7. Pistachio Pudding

Ingredients:

- Low-potassium instant pistachio pudding mix
- Low-potassium milk alternative
- Optional chopped pistachios

Instructions:

1. Make pistachio pudding according to package directions, substituting low-potassium milk.

2. Refrigerate until completely set.

3. If preferred, garnish with chopped pistachios.

Preparation Time: 15 Minutes

8. Lemon Sorbet

Ingredients:

- Lemon juice, freshly squeezed
- Lemon zest
- Optional sugar
- Water

Instructions:

1. Combine fresh lemon juice, lemon zest, and sugar (if using) in a saucepan.

2. Cook until the sugar melts.

3. Allow the mixture to cool before adding water.

4. Freeze until hard, or serve right away.

Preparation Time: 20 minutes

9. Raisin Oatmeal Cookies

Ingredients:

- Oatmeal
- Raisins
- Wheat flour
- Coconut oil
- Optional: maple syrup

Instructions:

1. Preheat the oven to 350°F. In a mixing bowl, combine the oats, raisins, whole wheat flour, coconut oil, and maple syrup (if using).

2. Bake the cookies till golden brown.

Preparation Time: 20 minutes

10. Mango Sorbet

Ingredients:

Mango chunks, frozen

Lime juice

Optional agave syrup

Instructions:

1. In a blender, combine frozen mango chunks and lime juice until smooth.

2. If more sweetness is wanted, add agave syrup.

3. Freeze until hard, or serve right now.

Preparation Time: 15 Minutes

10 Smoothies:

1. Smoothie with Berry Bliss

Ingredients:

- 1/2 cup fresh blueberries
- 1/2 cup hulled strawberries
- 1/2 cup fresh raspberries
- 1 cup yogurt with reduced potassium
- Cubes of ice

Instructions:

1. Puree blueberries, strawberries, raspberries, low-potassium yogurt, and ice cubes in a food processor until smooth.

2. Pour into a glass and drink up!

Preparation Time: 10 minutes

2. Mango Mint Delight

Ingredients:

- 1 cup mango chunks, frozen
- Half a banana
- 1 tablespoon mint leaves, fresh
- 1 cup coconut water (low potassium)
- Cubes of ice

Instructions:

1. Blend until smooth frozen mango chunks, banana, fresh mint leaves, low-potassium coconut water, and ice cubes.

2. Pour into a glass and enjoy the light flavors.

Preparation Time: 10 minutes

3. Smoothie with Cucumber Melon

Ingredients:

- 1/2 peeled and sliced cucumber
- 1 cup cubed honeydew melon
- 1/2 cup yogurt with reduced potassium
- Mint leaves for decoration
- Cubes of ice

Instructions:

1. Puree the cucumber, honeydew melon, low-potassium yogurt, and ice cubes in a blender until smooth.

2. Garnish with fresh mint leaves and serve chilled.

Preparation Time: 15 Minutes

4. Smoothie with Pineapple Basil Bliss

Ingredients:

- 1 cup pineapple cubes
- Half a banana
- 1 tablespoon basil leaves, fresh
- 1 cup almond milk (low in potassium)
- Cubes of ice

Instructions:

1. Puree the pineapple chunks, banana, fresh basil leaves, low-potassium almond milk, and ice cubes in a food processor until smooth.

2. Pour into a glass and enjoy the tropical treat.

Preparation Time: 10 minutes

5. Green Goddess Smoothie

Ingredients:

- a handful of spinach leaves
- half an avocado
- 1/2 cup sliced cucumber
- 1 cup coconut water (low potassium)
- Cubes of ice

Instructions:

1. Puree spinach leaves, avocado, cucumber, low-potassium coconut water, and ice cubes in a food processor until smooth.

2. Strain into a glass and enjoy the nutrient-dense bliss.

Preparation Time: 10 minutes

6. Smoothie with Papaya and Passion

Ingredients:

- 1 cup chunked papaya
- 1/2 cup chunked mango
- 1/2 cup Greek yogurt (low in potassium)
- 1 teaspoon chia seeds
- Cubes of ice

Instructions:

1. Puree the papaya, mango, low-potassium Greek yogurt, chia seeds, and ice cubes until smooth.

2. Pour the tropical fusion into a glass and drink.

Preparation Time: 10 minutes

7. Smoothie with Apple Pie

Ingredients:

- 1 cored and sliced apple
- 1/2 teaspoon cinnamon
- 1/4 teaspoon ground nutmeg
- 1 cup oat milk with low potassium
- Cubes of ice

Instructions:

1. Puree apple slices, cinnamon, nutmeg, low-potassium oat milk, and ice cubes in a food processor until smooth.

2. Pour into a glass and enjoy the apple pie flavor in a nutritious smoothie.

Preparation Time: 10 minutes

8. Cherry Almond Euphoria

Ingredients:

- 1/2 cup pitted cherries
- 1/4 cup sliced almonds
- 1 cup rice milk (low in potassium)
- 1 tbsp honey (optional).
- Cubes of ice

Instructions:

1. Puree cherries, almonds, low-potassium rice milk, honey (if using), and ice cubes in a food processor until smooth.

2. Pour into a glass and enjoy the delectable combo.

Preparation Time: 10 minutes

9. Carrot Cake Smoothie

Ingredients:

- 1/2 cup peeled and sliced carrots
- Half a banana
- 1 tablespoon cinnamon
- 1 cup coconut water (low potassium)

- Cubes of ice

Instructions:

1. Puree carrots, banana, cinnamon, low-potassium coconut water, and ice cubes in a food processor until smooth.

2. Pour into a glass and enjoy the flavor of carrot cake in a nutritious smoothie.

Preparation Time: 10 minutes

10. Smoothie with Pomegranate Paradise

Ingredients:

- pomegranate seeds, 1/2 cup
- Half a cup pineapple pieces
- 1/2 cup yogurt with reduced potassium
- 1 tbsp flaxseeds
- Cubes of ice

Instructions:

1. In a blender, combine the pomegranate seeds, pineapple chunks, low-fat yogurt, flaxseeds, and ice cubes until smooth.

2. Strain into a glass and enjoy the unusual flavors.

Preparation Time: 10 minutes

While Adhering To A Low-potassium Diet For Seniors, These Recipes Offer A Range Of Flavors. Adjust The Component Quantities As Needed And Speak With A Healthcare Expert Or Dietitian To Verify They Are Compatible With Specific Health Conditions And Nutritional Needs.

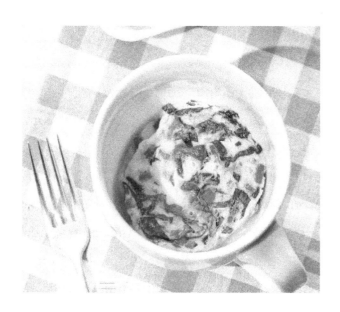

CONCLUSION

Finally, adopting a low-potassium diet for seniors can considerably improve their general health. This cookbook sought to give a varied selection of delectable and nutritionally balanced meals geared to seniors with potassium limits. The dishes stress delectable alternatives without sacrificing health, from breakfast to dinner, snacks to desserts. Seniors can enjoy a fulfilling culinary experience while following to their dietary requirements by combining inventive food replacements, portion control, and attentive meal planning. It is critical to seek tailored advice from healthcare specialists or nutritionists. Adopting a low-potassium lifestyle not only benefits specific health concerns, but it also promotes a more holistic approach to senior nutrition, boosting vitality and fostering a higher quality of life. May this cookbook encourage a path toward delectable and healthy options that enable seniors to prioritize their health while also enjoying the pleasures of good eating.

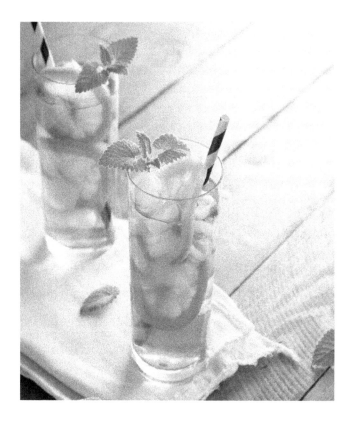